Bad Days

Build

Better Days

A guide on how to break through the break downs.

By Casey Blum

No part of this publication may be reproduced, stored in a retrieval system, or transmitted in any form or by any means, electronic, photocopying, recording, or otherwise without prior written permission, except in the case of brief excerpts in critical reviews and articles. For permission requests, contact the author at Caseyfitcakes@gmail.com

Copyright © 2019 Casey Blum

ISBN: 9781701621053

The author disclaims responsibility for adverse effects or consequences from misapplication or injudicious use of the information contained in this book. Mention of resources and association does not imply an endorsement. If you are experiencing a mental health crisis reach out to a doctor or use the National Suicide Prevention hotline 1-800-273-8255.

I am not a professional, this book is not meant to take place of medical help. I am just sharing my story in hopes to inspire you to make a change.

Preface

"You were assigned this mountain to show others it can

be moved"

-Mel Robbins

There's been numerous times in my life where I've questioned God. I would wonder why the heck this is happening to ME!? What did I ever do to deserve this misfortune and pain? There were a lot of times I didn't think I'd make it through anymore. I was always blaming others for my pain and stuck in victim mode.

It took me a long time, (about 24 years) to be able to see the positive in things. To know that things don't just happen *to* me, but *for me* and I can take it with a grain of salt and move on or I can let it break me.

I believe everyone in this world was created for a reason, you all have a job to make an impact in this world, whatever that may be! I believe I had to hit my breaking point and go through some tough stuff in my life so I could write this book for you and realize what my reason was. I am going to share with you my breaking point that all started back in 2015... it's still very hard to write this out.

There I was standing on this mountain 10,000 feet up, looking down thinking I could just end it all right now. I remember thinking to myself, "nobody would even notice that I'm gone, I don't have a purpose here I make coffee for a living" and those thoughts haunted me for the 4 hour climb back down and the next 2 years while I battled to stay alive.

I was sliding down this mountain, because you shouldn't wear Nikes that don't have traction to climb a 13-mile mountain. As I was sliding down, I didn't really care if I slid off the mountain or not, and that's a really scary and sad thing to think. To not care if you died, to not be afraid of death. I had never felt this way before and it scared me. When I got off the mountain 8 hours later, I realized that I just battled my first suicide thought. I had never felt this way before and I wasn't sure if I'd ever feel it again but all I know is that mountain just changed my life more than I ever thought possible.

A day later I went and got a tattoo of mountains and the word "live" on my wrist. I don't know why I just felt compelled to do so, I didn't even have the money to do it I was very broke. I lived off of bagels and lemon poppyseed muffin tops from the coffee shop I worked at for that week. I went through very hard times for almost two years, little did I know I would face suicidal thoughts many more times.

Fast forward four years later and I'm writing this from a beautiful house, my boyfriend and I got together. I get to choose every day if I want to work from my bed, office, or the coffee shop down the road. We have two blue heelers, my dream dogs with a huge backyard for them to run around and my favorite place to hike just down a back road. I'm with a man who wants to build a future with me and works so hard every day to provide and love me. We have money in savings, and I get to make an impact on women's lives every single day with my business. It's crazy how life works out.

This was all a dream to me that I never thought would happen, I was willing to just stop everything and give up my life because I didn't think things would get any better. But here I am living my dream and feeling truly happy.

I haven't struggled with depression for almost a year now, the last time was because I lost my best friend in a car accident. I did this without the help of drugs. Although I know everyone is different and drugs do help people, I'm going to share my story and how I changed my life around without them. The power of taking control of your mindset can be an amazing thing.

I hope this can help you if you're in the same spot I was four years ago. I know it feels like everything sucks and you want to be done with it all, but I promise you-

Bad days build better days.

In Honor of....

Mary Guynn
1/23/95-08/10/18

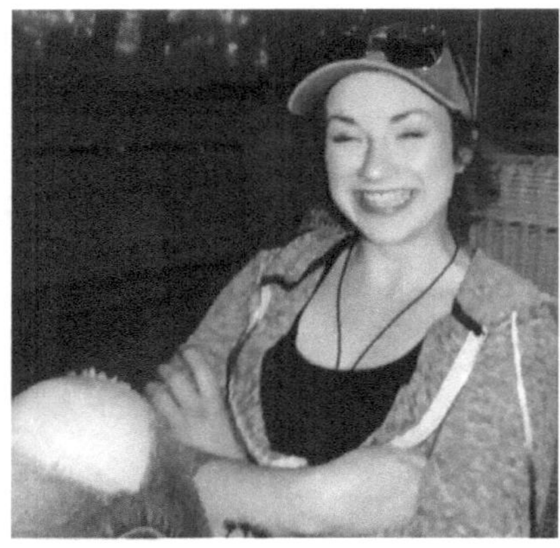

Your love, words, and laugh were such a bright light for so many. You were

taken from us way too soon. In the 23 years you were here you saved so many

from the unthinkable and never let it shake you. I hope that I can take the

love you shared with me on my darkest days freshmen year and give it to
others who need it.

I hope this book can continue to be your bright light Mary.

Table of Contents

Preface *3*

In Honor of…. *6*

Bad Days Build Better Days *8*

The First Step to Living *1*

The Second Step to Living *4*

The Third Step to Living *8*

The Fourth Step to Living *12*

The Fifth Step to Living *15*

The Sixth Step to Living *19*

The Seventh Step to Living *23*

The Eighth Step to Living *26*

The Ninth Step to Living *29*

The Tenth Step to Living *33*

Bad Days Build Better Days

It can be easy to think that some people have life figured out. That just because they know exactly what they want to do, and they have the money to get there (or their parents support) they go to school, get their stuff paid for, and even drive a nice car. It may seem like on the outside that they don't ever have to struggle. The truth is though, everyone struggles. Rather they have to check their bank account for every purchase or not, everyone is fighting some kind of mental battle. They may have it all and have everything together on the outside, but their world might be falling apart on the inside.

When I first starting writing this book, (which by the way was just a blog post at the time) I thought I was the ONLY one who fought inner demons and then I realized there are so many more people like me and probably you since you're reading this book who have been through hell and *keep* pushing. The people who don't get handed things in life, who have to work hard for everything and still feel like we have nothing. The people who DO have the anxiety attacks on their bathrooms floors every day, but then have to pull it together and put a smile on their face for work. The ones who can't afford groceries so you pick up more shifts at work, even though you just worked every day since who knows when and you can't even catch a break. The ones who just want to disappear, but nobody would ever guess.

<u>You are the strongest person I know.</u>

It's hard to live life like that. But you are the person they write books about. You are the person who gets the standing ovation because life is hard, especially when doing it alone and here you are still living and breathing.

I know it may not seem like it now, but I promise you... life will get so much better.

Bad days build better days and I'm going to show you how.

I'm going to show you how I went from stressed, depressed, and literally no money even while working 80-hour weeks to sitting in my apartment making 6 figures.

This never would have happened if I listened to my inner demons four years ago on that mountain, it also would have never happened if I didn't have that breaking point in my life. I thank South Sister every day for that moment. It made me stronger and it made me learn how to live the life I wanted.

If you want to break out of this dark hole, then turn the page.

If you're not ready to get real with yourself and put in the work, then put this book down.

I promise you it will be hard, but it will be worth it.

The First Step to Living

I will list out what you need to do by chapter.

The first step is visualization. Now before you roll your eyes at me, just hear me out. What's life without dreaming of what you want? You can't just go through the motions every day- you need to have a goal in mind that shapes the actions you do every day.

So, what do you want your life to be?

Get out a piece of paper and pen and start brain dumping.

If you could live anywhere in the world what place brings up the most happiness when you think about it?

If you could have any job, what would it be? Why does it make you feel that way? Are you happy with your current job? What would you change?

If you could own anything, what would you get? Why? How would that make you happier than you are now?

What would you do on a daily basis when you get to this spot in your life?

What makes you happy?

Go on… list everything I just mentioned here. Look, I've read tons of these books where they say, "create a list" and you're like, "okay whatever Karen it's in my head" … but I SWEAR TO YOU there is power in writing this stuff down. The fact that you take time to go find paper and a pen and write this down, means you're ready to make a change, my friend.

Look, if you skip this exercise like I use to then you might as well throw the book away. The only way I can help you is if you do the mindset work.

To prove you are really ready for a change email me at Caseyfitcakes@gmail.com and say "I am ready for a change" this is my personal email, I'll reply! No annoying automation or spam, just person to person support.

Take time to journal about this last chapter:

The Second Step to Living

So, the first step was to visualize what you want to happen in your life. Now the next step is to make it happen. To create goals that you're so passionate about accomplishing you'll give up everything to achieve.

Not everyone is driven by a goal and not everyone is motivated! So, this is why we need a bigger outcome, a bigger picture for you.

Picture what it would feel and be like if you were to achieve this goal of yours.

Say your goal was to live in Hawaii. How would it feel to walk out your door onto the sandy warm beaches knowing this wasn't just some vacation? You had beach hair, tanned skin, and drank coffee at the local beach hut down the road.

How would that make you feel?

Now hold onto that emotion. That feeling is going to get you through the hardest days, because you know the end is going to be worth it all.

I want you to take all the visualizations you wrote down for your life and find pictures that fit those and print them out and TAPE THEM TO YOUR WALL. Find pictures that gives you that giddy, warm heart feeling like a kid trying to sleep on Christmas Eve. That way your goals are no longer just "something you want to accomplish" you are looking at a picture of it every day and it's bringing emotion to you that makes you motivated and excited!

This can be for ANYTHING. You can make goals in your life for whatever, it's just important to have something to work for.

My vision board last year looked like:

Pictures of Colorado because I wanted to live there, a cute picture of a couple in a tent because I wanted to find someone who I love and would go backpacking with me, a blue heeler puppy, a jeep, a model I look up to and find her body to be inspiration for myself, and a super cute gym because I can't wait to open my own!

I looked at all every single day and it motivated me, some seem silly or simple like a blue heeler puppy. Dogs are expensive and take a lot of work and I just didn't have the time at the moment but I was working my butt off in my business so I could have the freedom to have one... Now I have two!

Think about the last time you set goals or maybe you just said something like, "I'm going to lose 10 pounds" and it quickly disappeared from your mind.

Maybe you were motivated for a little, but then life got busy and you got tired, so you forgot about your goals. It happens. But not when you're looking at it every day! When you're staring at your goals and a little glimpse of what your future could look like if you just kept pushing through.

That is what will keep you motivated during the hard times.

Remember that the goal is to get a little bit better each day.

List what you need to do to accomplish these life goals. Create a game plan! How much money do you need? What do you need to do to get there? Maybe it's hiring a trainer or a life coach. Pick up another job if you need to. Tell your friends and family to keep you accountable and make these goals come to life!

Take time to journal about this last chapter:

The Third Step to Living

You have to change your mindset.

You know when you're sick or having a bad mental health day. You just want to get some ice cream or soup and lay in bed all day? You just want to sit in that crappy feeling and almost feel bad for yourself because doing something good for yourself sounds like a lot of work.

Well sister, you need to get out of bed and do the things that will actually make you feel good. I read a book by Rachel Hollis called "Girl, Wash Your Face" I HIGHLY suggest this book, but I wanted to tell you about it because just the title is so powerful. So, girl… get up and wash your dang face. Feel the cold water on you and put on a good moisturizer and get to rocking.

You have to learn how to kick yourself out of these ruts. It won't be easy and sometimes you won't win, but you need to try. You can start learning how to switch your mindset and change your feelings in little ways like for an example, when you're driving, and someone cuts you off or does something stupid that would make you mad and want to flip them off…. Smile at them! Right there you're training your brain to find the positive instead of negative. There's power in being able to control your emotions. It will help you on your hardest days.

Having the ability to change your mindset when you start to fade into a bad day will help you turn everything around.

It's all about the law of attraction and manifestation! The Law of Attraction states that if you want something good or positive to happen in your life, you have to think positively. However, if you think negatively you more than likely will have negative outcomes in life. It sounds weird but it's the truth.

How many times have you had a bad day and then you're constantly saying, "wow today is so awful, what else could go wrong?" AND THEN something else happens!! Well, The Law of Attraction says that we attract what we put out. So, if you're constantly putting out negative vibes, negative things will continue to happen, and you'll just fall into this cycle of "when will this day ever end".

When you have a positive outlook EVEN when things go wrong, it just feels better and gets better. Your attitude not only affects what comes your way, but everyone around you. You can tell, literally feel, when someone has a bad vibe to them. So, change your mindset and vibrate at a higher, more positive frequency.

Manifestation works the same, as your thoughts control your actions. If you're telling yourself every day how much your life sucks and how unhappy you are, odds are it's going to continue to be crappy. But if you tell yourself things like how amazing your life is and how you're so successful and living in abundance, you'll feel better and start to live that way. The truth is our brains don't know the difference between a lie and the truth. So, if you tell yourself the things you want to be true and you start to believe them, they will become reality.

I have these "Pain-to-Power" examples written down and taped to my bathroom mirror as a constant reminder! I highly suggest you write them down and put them somewhere you can see all the time.

Pain --> **Power**

I can't ……………………………………………………. I won't

I should…………………………...…………………………...I could

It's not my fault…………………………………. I'm totally responsible

It's a problem……………………………...…………………It's an opportunity

I'm never satisfied………………...…..…………..I want to learn and grow

Life's a struggle……………………………….……...Life's an adventure

I hope…………………………………………….…………… I know

If only………………………...…………………………...Next time

What will I do?..I know I can handle it

It's terrible…………………….…....................It's a learning experience

Take time to journal about this last chapter:

____

____

____

____

____

____

____

____

____

The Fourth Step to Living

Get your booty into gear.

Find your form of "fitness" and get to moving. According to an article found on WebMD by <u>Smitha Bhandari, MD</u> "When you work out, your body releases endorphins which interact with the receptors in your brain that reduce your perception of pain. Endorphins also trigger a positive feeling in the body, that's what people call "runners high" you can actually get a more positive outlook on life or feel happier from just exercising for 30 minutes a day."

Exercise can be done in many ways! You could go to the gym and lift weights, go for a walk, hike, bike riding, swimming, a dance class, yoga, or a group fitness class.

I highly suggest getting involved in a group class setting. Something you have to pay for and if you don't make it to the class, you don't get your money back. See if you can find someone to go with you or make a friend in the class and hold each other accountable! You won't always feel like going so when you have money or someone to keep you accountable, you'll be more likely to commit.

Group settings are also great for many reasons: it forces you out of your comfort zone to work out and interact with different people. You might even push yourself harder seeing everyone around you.

There are lots of Facebook Groups or the app "Meetup" that you can find "your people" to go do things with! Hiking groups, biking, or even book clubs. Push yourself to find your tribe and meet new people every day.

Social media has made it very easy to share your story and connect with likeminded people. Even if you already have some amazing friends, I think it's very important to meet new people.

If you prefer to be in a gym setting but you don't know what to do, then hire a trainer. A lot of gyms offer a free session, so you can learn a routine and stick to it. You don't need to do something new every day. YouTube, Bodybuilding.com, Instagram, or my website (caseyfitcakes.com) are great resources for this. I've been a trainer for four years, but it wasn't always like that.

I used to be afraid of the gym and nervous of what people would think. I would sit in the bathroom and YouTube a workout plan or how to use a machine so nobody would see me confused in the gym. I was 50 pounds overweight and not the slightest clue of what "nutrition" was.

Until I hired a trainer.

I thank fitness every day for saving my life. The gym gave me an outlet on my hard days, when I was stressed or upset, I could just turn up the music and go workout. It taught me that my body needed more than just McDonald's, Taco bell, and Red bull to function. It taught me that I'd rather be up early on a Saturday working out than hung over.

Through my weight loss journey, I gained my life.

And maybe you don't have any weight to lose. You are happy with how your body looks, which is great!! But there's still so many benefits that working out can bring. So, I really suggest you find what you love to do and then do it regularly. It takes a while to make exercise a habit, keep pushing through even on the days you don't feel like going because one day it'll be what you look forward to!

Take time to journal about this last chapter:

The Fifth Step to Living

You have to realize that nobody else is going to make you happy. No friend, family member, or relationship can change how you feel and make you truly happy on the inside. Sure, there are people that make us feel good and bring happiness to our life. But at the end of the day you need to face your demons and be able to be fully happy with yourself.

You can tell when someone is not happy with themselves. It comes out in insecurities and rage towards others.

Jealousy, controlling, manipulation, clingy, needy, procrastinating, lack of confidence, etc.

Not being happy with yourself will cause problems in your relationships, every kind, and will hold you back in your life.

How are you supposed to accomplish everything on your dream board if you are not confident in yourself? If you don't know your worth!?

Now being happy with yourself is a never-ending journey! It's not like you can just look in the mirror and say, "okay

I'm happy now!" This has been something I have been learning for a long time.

Here are some things I realized became habits when I wasn't happy in myself and maybe you see yourself forming these habits too;

I was drinking a lot due to lack of confidence, anytime I was at a social event I needed to have a buzz to fit in and feel comfortable.

I had very surface level relationships, I basically just had drinking buddies and constantly felt alone.

I was single for a good chunk of time, which is no problem but anytime I did meet a guy I found myself running into the biggest jerks because that's what I was attracting into my life.

I made bare minimum in my jobs and I did the very bare minimum in them to get by. I also accumulated a lot of debt and was not smart with my money.

Now these are all habits that form when you don't care to grow. I was just going through the motions every day and doing what I needed to get by in life. I know that's not what you want any more though because you are reading this book, you are ready for change.

So, these are the daily tasks I do to make sure I feel good and to love myself more and to grow into the person I want to be:

Practice some sort of self-development every day, this can be reading a book, listening to a podcast, or attending a seminar

Take care of your body every day with movement, we aren't meant to be stagnant, so go for a walk, a hike, a workout, anything to move for at least 30 minutes.

Eat things that will make you feel good and not like garbage, so next time you find yourself in the Taco Bell line at 3pm on a Tuesday rethink your actions.

Surround yourself with the kind of people you want to be. You should always walk away from a time with your friends feeling uplifted and happy, not drained.

Limit alcohol (or drug) intake. Stop trying to escape reality! It's okay every once in a while, like when you're at an event. But see how you feel on a daily basis without these suppressants in your life.

Incorporating these small habits have made a huge impact in my life. See we as humans are creatures of routine. We don't realize but EVERYTHING we do on a daily basis is because of habits we have established. Like brushing your teeth when you wake up and go to sleep (or maybe you don't lol) that is a habit we formed when we were little, sometimes we don't even realize we are doing it-we just do. Your whole day is formed of habits. So, take some time to reflect and think if those habits are setting you up for success or holding you back.

Take time to journal about this last chapter:

The Sixth Step to Living

Eliminate any negativity. I'm not just talking people- if there's anything that doesn't bring you an abundance of joy, walk away. A job? School? Relationship/Friendship? GO.

I promise you as cliché as it sounds: when one door closes, another one will open. But you can't achieve new opportunities if you're holding onto things that bring you down.

Think about it, when you're stressed/upset BAD THINGS KEEP HAPPENING!! It's like what the heck life, when can you catch a break!? That's how it is when you have things in your life bringing you negativity. Like maybe your friend group likes to sit around and talk about people, you just sit there, and they scroll through social media and bag on everyone that pops up. Or maybe you go into work every day dreading it because it's such a toxic situation (we all know what I'm talking about) maybe your boss is a jerk and you get anxious anytime he walks into the room because you never know what he'll get mad about now, or maybe you work in customer service and your customers are rude! Maybe you're in school and maybe you even don't want to be in school, but your parents really want you to be. So, you work hard in class every day, but you dread it so much and studying is sucking the life out of you and you don't even want to be learning this stuff. Or you have a relationship that is not building you up and making you feel good, you feel trapped and "icky", but you don't know how you'll live without them.

All of those are hard situations. You may feel stuck whatever situation you're in right now, but I promise you are NOT. Literally there is nothing holding you back. You can do whatever the heck you want (as long as you're 18 of course otherwise your parents do have a say.). If something is not bringing happiness into your life, L.E.A.V.E literally run now. Put in your two weeks notice, break up with the douchebag, blow off your crappy friends for new ones, drop out of school. These all sound like "icky" things to do but they are SO FREEING. Why would you ever live your life unhappy? There is seriously so much out there in this huge world, I promise you will find a new job, find amazing friends, maybe find a new major in school or a career without it, and especially you will find someone who loves you and doesn't make you feel worthless.

I don't just preach this; I live this to full extent too. In the last 9 years I've had 32 jobs I always giggle a little when I say that because the look on people's faces are like WHAT SERIOUSLY. The longest I've ever kept a job is 2 years and that was at a coffee shop, Dutch Bros but technically I moved towns and stands so it was like a year each. I learned at a young age that I will never stay in a situation that doesn't bring me happiness. Maybe I adopted this from my childhood. I watched my parents fight constantly. In fact, I never once saw them love on each other it was very sad but mostly for them. I knew they weren't happy, and I actually encouraged a divorce. It wasn't fair that they stayed together when they were miserable, both of them deserved happiness. So, I think now I'm afraid that if I ever stay in a situation that doesn't make me happy, that I will be stuck. I know that's not a life I ever want myself or anyone to live.

So, any job that I didn't "love" or feel happy with, I quit. Usually right on the spot because within a couple weeks or months I could tell if it would serve me or not. Any relationship friend or significant other if I didn't feel love and abundance from, I'd cut off. I'm a college dropout X3 I kept trying different majors in different times of my life, but it just wasn't for me!

And you know what, that is okay. It's okay to know what makes you happy and what doesn't serve you. I've had a lot of people tell me "you just have commitment issues" no, no, no I just know what I want in life.

Maybe you are unsure of what is bringing you down in your life. You know something feels off but you're just not sure what it is.

I encourage you to grab a piece of paper and write down everything you're doing right now and the name of every person you spend time with. Now you're going to sit there and one by one read off what's on your paper, think about how that makes you feel. If you read off your job what is your first initial reaction? Do you feel good or do you dread it? (I promise people do actually love their job it's possible so if you don't, keep searching)

Now read off the names of the people you spend the most time with, how do they make you feel? Are you happy they are in your life or is there some mixed emotions? They say that you are a reflection of the 5 people you spend the most time around.

Maybe it's where you live or what you do on a daily basis? Whatever it is get down to the root of the problem and make some changes. If you're dealing with a friendship that isn't making you feel good, but you really value that friendship then talk to them. Let them know how you feel and that you want things to change, if they don't understand then cut it off. It's HARD. But take it from someone who lost both of her closest best friends of 7 years. You can live without them and you will make new friends, it will be very hard, but you will be just fine. It's been over a year since I lost one of my best friends in a car accident and the other from a stupid fight. I am okay.

Take time to journal about this last chapter:

The Seventh Step to Living

Eliminate anything, any substance that makes you escape reality.

Think about it- what do you do when you get home after a long day? What do you crave when you're really stressed out? Do you reach for a drink, a smoke, a cookie, a shopping spree? What are you using to cope and cover up emotions? Maybe you don't realize you are, just like I did. I thought it was normal to want to have a beer after a long week, something to take the edge off and make me feel better. We normalize this stuff so much that you probably thought uh yeah everyone does that! But really you are masking some sort of emotion that you need to deal with.

For instance, have you ever gone through a breakup or something that really upset you and then you went out with all your girlfriends and you didn't mean to, but you drank WAY too much and now you're in the bathroom crying? It's because you finally felt emotions that you didn't allow yourself to completely feel at the time when you were sober, instead you went and drank and now they are pouring out of you.

This happens a lot in life if you're not completely in tune with your thoughts and emotions you may be covering up a lot that one day and then drunk or not it will come pouring out. So, I challenge you to go 30 days without whatever you use to "make you feel better" this isn't just alcohol. It can be watching Netflix when you're sad, so you don't have to think about your thoughts, stress eating sweets, smoking any substance, maybe even sexual relationships. Whatever your go to is I want you to cut it out for 30 days.

Maybe you don't realize what you are doing to mask any emotions, if so, I want you to grab a journal (Target run!!) and start writing down your thoughts EVERY DAY. This is going to help you understand how you are feeling and how you can change things.

Journaling Prompt:

How am I feeling today? (write down every emotion that comes to mind)

I feel anxious today and a little stressed out about money. There's just so many bills to be paid, it seems like I can't catch a break.

And then flip your script:

I feel amazing today, I am living in so much abundance. I am so happy I have the money to pay these bills in order for me to live. I have a roof over my head, a working phone, and food. That is more than a lot of people have. Today is a great day!

So, I just took my anxious feelings and poured all this positivity into my mind. Remember, your mind doesn't know the difference between a truth and a lie. Tell yourself the things you want to hear. If you feel anxious and depressed, write it down and then flip the script and make yourself feel good. I promise you this works! Try it every day.

Use the journaling pages at the end of the book if you don't want to go buy a journal! I make this very easy for you.

Take time to journal about this last chapter:

The Eighth Step to Living

Now that we've talked about eliminating all the negativity and toxic thoughts let's figure out what lights your soul on fire. This was the key step to getting me through my darkest days and still helps me, you need to find something worth living for. Something that makes you jump out of bed because you're so excited.

So many of my days were spent wondering what I was living for. It felt like all I did was worked and then drank a lot of beers and went to sleep. I truly believe every single person in this world has a purpose; I just couldn't find mine, for a while. It wasn't until I stepped foot into a gym that my whole entire world changed. I went through a weight loss journey and with the weight I lost I had no clue that I would gain my life back. One day something clicked, and I decided that I was going to be a personal trainer so I could teach other women how to do this and feel good about themselves. So, I paid for a course that I did not have the money for (thank you credit cards) and started my journey to where I am now.

Now I wake up every day so eager to do what I do; I found my purpose in the oddest of ways. I change women's lives daily. I still can't wrap my mind around this! That ME, lil ole' depressed me that wanted to end her life, that worked at a coffee shop with no direction, that couldn't even pay her bills because she was too broke from the bars, CHANGING LIVES. Wow. Seriously girlfriend, if I can do it, you can too. This is exactly how you're going to figure out what lights up your soul.

You get out into the world and you do the things that are uncomfortable. Because, growth and good things don't come to those who confine themselves into a little box called their comfort zone. Sign up for that class, go to the meetup group, message someone on social media to hang out. Just do it! I know it's scary I still get cold feet when I'm about to join a new group, but you do it anyways and you need to continue to go. There is so much opportunity out in the world just waiting for you. You just need to put your big girl pants on and go get it. Sign up for a new yoga class and actually go to the classes, get comfortable there, smile at people and make small talk, then after a couple classes start actually introducing yourself like "Hey I'm Casey, I've seen you here a couple times and just wanted to introduce myself!"

There are endless classes you can do! Exercise, hiking, rock climbing, pottery, painting, guitar, cooking, book clubs ...I could go on for days. Point is to find something that interests you and go! That is where you will find your tribe, because you are doing something you enjoy and trust me you never know what can come of it!

Facebook groups, Bumble BFF, and Meetup are great ways to find these classes or your new friends. It's going to feel scary, but you have to get out there. You have to break free of your normal routine to see what else life has for you. I would never be where I am now if I kept working overtime at a coffee shop and staying till closing time at the bars every weekend. Amazing things and opportunities are coming your way.

Take time to journal about this last chapter:

The Ninth Step to Living

Loving the atmosphere you are in, this ties in with everything I've been talking about in the last couple of chapters. Nothing is worse than living somewhere or working somewhere that you don't love and that isn't serving you. I've already talked about how toxic a work environment can be if you don't enjoy it, but now I want to dive into your home, the place you probably spend the majority of your time at, your "safe space".

First, think about- do you like where you are living? Are you living with roommates that bug you (been there, it sucks) or maybe with your parents? Or maybe you just don't like the area you are in.

Whatever you don't like, I am giving you permission to leave. You might think okay but what about finding a new place or coming up with money for a deposit!? It will all work out; you just need to start creating a plan. I've broken many leases, paid for apartments that were way out of my budget, and even went to court with a landlord. I've lived in many spaces, good and bad..very bad. If you need any roommate or apartment hunting advice, I am your go-to girl. If you are living in a spot you are in right now that you don't enjoy you probably already know that it is a very draining feeling. Walking through the door of your home should put you at peace, you should be happy to come home. Not stressed out.

So, if you want to find a new place to live but you're stuck in a lease with a crappy roommate then here's what I suggest. Always be skimming Craigslist or Facebook for a new place, maybe someone who needs a roommate or get your own place. Keep in mind wherever you go you will need a deposit so start putting money aside for this. Be open with your roommate BUT ONLY when you have enough to cover a deposit probably $600-$1,000. tell them that things just aren't working out and you'd like to find another place to live and you will help fill your spot in the lease. Sometimes it goes well and sometimes it doesn't, but you need to make yourself a priority. They will figure things out!

If you like your living situation but it just doesn't bring you joy, then it's time for a deep clean and make over. I find myself rearranging furniture monthly. It feels so good to clean things up and move them around. Maybe go buy some new decor or a candle. In order to be happy and productive your space needs to be clean. You'll be surprised how much of a better mood you'll have when your space is dusted off and moved around.

If you are just sick of your town... MOVE. Nothing is holding you back, pick a spot on the map and load up what you can and figure it out. If it doesn't work out, you can always move back. This is the best thing I've ever done for myself, multiple times. At 20, I moved 3 hours from home and started a new life where I didn't know anyone, I learned a lot about myself and my relationships by doing this. Yes, it was scary, but it was much needed. I moved back home to regather myself after 3 years and then I took off for a road trip 23 hours away from home.

Oregon to Colorado with my doggie and boyfriend. We ended up hating it there, so we moved back home once again. Sometimes home is really where you belong, but you need to get out in the world and discover new things to know where you should be.

You need to start taking matters into your own hands and pretty much screw other people's opinions or feelings. When I knew I wanted to move to Colorado, my best friend of 8 years convinced me not to, she was so upset and kind of mad that I would move so far from her and our little family we created. I agreed with her even though I was only 23 and wanted to see more of the world, I stayed in the little town we grew up in.

She's no longer in my life, months after she convinced me not to go and that I was a workaholic and needed to focus more on family she left my life we haven't talked for a year. My point is that I was so worried about HER feelings that I didn't do the things in my life that I wanted to and, in the end, she wasn't even around anymore.

I had a very important person in my life tell me once that everything is **temporary**. This has clung to me since the day she told me because it is actually very true. Your friendships, relationships, work, money, the bad days- can all be gone in a second. So, YOU need to do what's best for you. Make a move, do whatever is going to make you feel the best.

Whatever is in the back of your mind, you need to make happen. It may actually suck and be nothing like you imagined, just like Colorado was for me. But guess what? You can always come back. You can always make another move until you find where you are happy.

Take time to journal about this last chapter:

The Tenth Step to Living

Sometimes, you can go through all of these steps, do all of the self-care, and still need extra help. I want you to know it's OKAY to go talk to someone, a therapist-someone who went to school and is registered to help you with how you're feeling.

Having a friend, family member, or significant other to talk to is always great and you should have that support from your loved ones but there's so much you can learn and overcome from talking to a therapist.

In my opinion every person should talk to a therapist. Everyone is dealing with something whether they are aware of it or not. A therapist can find where these emotions are coming from and help you understand and get through them. There's some social confusion about therapists, people think if you go to one then "something's really wrong with you" which is something we need to break and start talking more about, just like mental health issues.

There is nothing wrong with seeking help or even just someone to talk to. This doesn't make you any weaker or lesser of a person, in fact it makes you that much stronger. Seeking out help shows that you want to make a change but it's hard by yourself. Just like hiring a personal trainer, you know what you need to do but you just can't sum up the motivation to do it yourself. You just need a push in the right direction.

Everyone in my family has seen a therapist including myself and it's helped everyone immensely. For a while I was nervous to go to a therapist, I'd tell myself "I can do this on my own, I don't need to waste time and money" they even have online therapists that you can do a skype or phone call session with and a lot of insurances will cover it. If money is your issue just think of this as an investment in your life and your health. Stop buying coffee every morning or new clothes for a month and you'll have enough to cover a couple of therapy sessions.

Just do what you need to do to take care of yourself. Buying this book was the first step and I hope it helped you, I hope that you share it with someone in need and that it helps them. Even if someone isn't suicidal, it just gives you a better and positive outlook on life. I wanted to create something that could help anyone even if they just have a couple of off days. I know a lot of people who silently struggle, a lot of people reach out to me because I make it known that I struggle through this so that people like you DON'T FEEL ALONE. I literally never get any pity messages, that's not what I want anyways, I only ever get messages of people saying, "wow I really needed this". So, I encourage you if you want to be a light in someone's life to give this book away and share your story, share your struggles. It's hard and scary but knowing that you could be helping someone else is worth it.

In case you ever feel like you're alone I just wanted to share some statistics that honestly gave me goosebumps. As of 2017, 300 million people in the world were DIAGNOSED with depression, meaning they went to the doctor and were diagnosed with depression. I know so many people who are depressed or anxious but never actually went to a doctor, you don't need a professional to diagnose you with something you can feel so hard. I've known since I was 12. Which leads me to the next heart-breaking statistic, suicide is the 2nd leading cause of death in ages from 10-34. Our children are depressed before they even know what it means, and you know where they are getting that from? Us. The parents. It rubs off in your everyday actions.

So, start talking, make some FREAKIN NOISE! Talk about your struggles and ask people how they are feeling.

Love on everyone. Take care of yourself. And remember,

Bad Days Build Better Days.

With all the love in the world,

Casey Marie

I just wanted to leave a place where you can message me if you ever need anything.

You can find me on Instagram at: Caseyfitcakes

Or my inbox is always open for you and that is: Caseyfitcakes@gmail.com

Please don't ever hesitate to reach out to me.

Extra pages to journal with: